the DEA STASH AND HIDEOUT HANDBOOK

The D.E.A. Stash and Hideout Handbook

ISBN 0-87364-469-7
Printed in the United States of America

Published by Paladin Press, a division of
Paladin Enterprises, Inc., P.O. Box 1307,
Boulder, Colorado 80306, USA.
(303) 443-7250

Direct inquiries and/or orders to the above address.

Illustrations courtesy of Bill Border

CONTENTS

The ***DEA Stash and Hideout Handbook*** was obtained via covert means from the U.S. Drug Enforcement Administration. This information has been classified "Top Secret -- Eyes Only" for DEA officers, and is information the DEA uses.

This is the actual list used in seminars conducted to train narcotics officers in search and seizure of drugs and contraband items. These seminars instruct many military, state, local, and foreign narcotics officers. The places listed here are not checked in every search, nor are these the only places searched.

Now you have the information that will help you either find someone else's stash or put your own where no one, not even many highly trained law-enforcement officers, will be able to find it!

We've all wondered from time to time, "Where would be a good, safe place to put my extra cash, my trusty firearm, or a valuable painting where no one will ever find it but me?" Wonder no longer. This list, used wisely, will put that valuable item beyond the reach of any save yourself.

The purpose of this list is to provide an insight into the mind of the searcher and to show the futility of hiding contraband under the socks in your dresser drawer. You *know* that putting cash in a vase on the dining room table or under the mattress of your bed is just plain crazy, and that hiding it under your pillow is not very wise either -- but where is a good place?

Consider the locations in your house that would most likely elude searching officers, K-9s, or criminals. From abandoned plumbing, under floor drains, and within tea bags to above acoustical tiles, behind wall and ceiling light fixtures, and inside shower nozzle heads.

Your car, motorcycle, and even your own body contain hundreds of unlikely hiding places, from the tiny spaces in jewelry, to the somewhat larger and much more private bodily cavities.

Although all these places are known to law enforcement agencies, many of them would serve quite well in most police searches. There are several trick stash containers on the market today, such as phony soft drink cans. This type of thing can prove very useful, and will fool all but the most determined of police.

But don't try to get these hide-outs past U.S. Customs officials -- they've seen them all!

INSIDE HOLLOW DOORS (REMOVABLE TOPS)

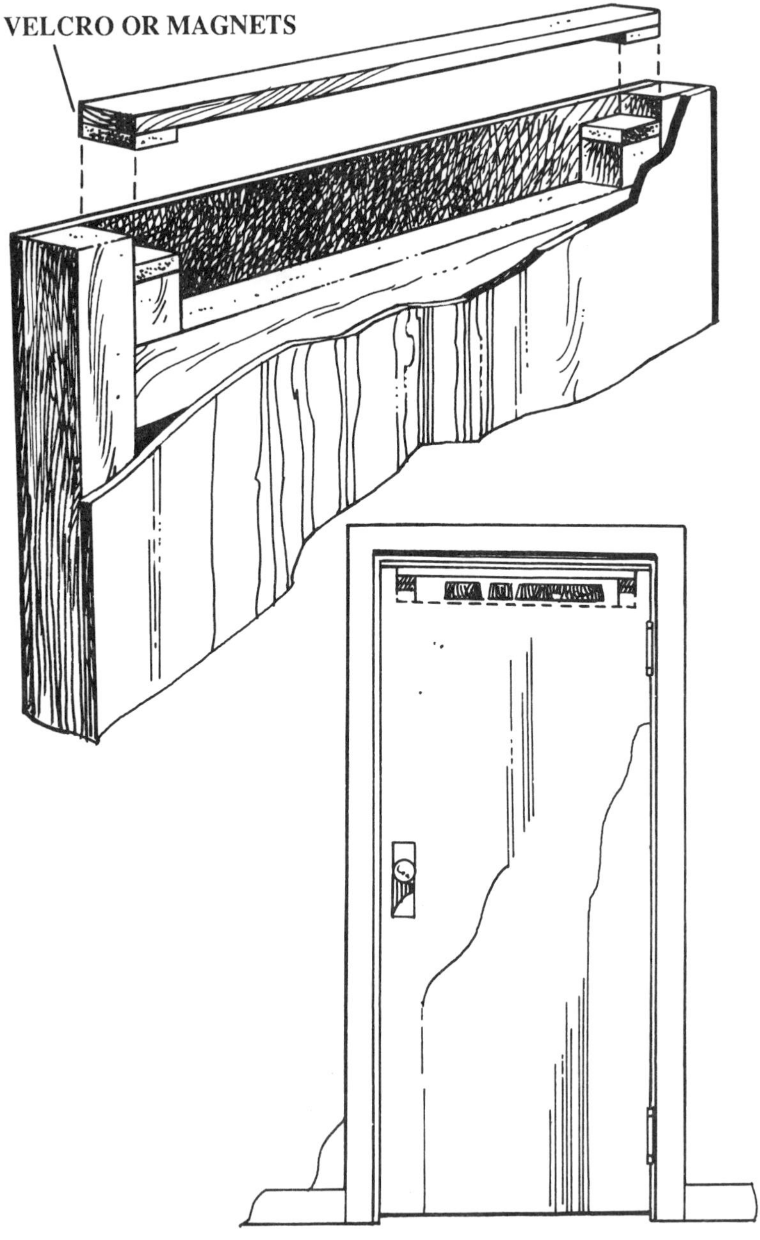

DRUG CONCEALMENT IN THE HOME

Under or in the mailbox
In flower pots and window boxes
Inside hollow doors (removable tops)
Inside door chimes and door bell
Behind plumbing inspection doors
In doorknobs
Under or in dog collars
Hanging out windows
In rolled-up window shades
On or under window ledge next door
On top of window, door sills, moldings
In fire and water hoses
In or on cellar beams
Taped to movable clothesline
Behind exterior brick near window
Inside fuse boxes
In conduit from fuse box
Inside fire alarm bell
In dog houses

IN TELEPHONE BASE AND HANDLE

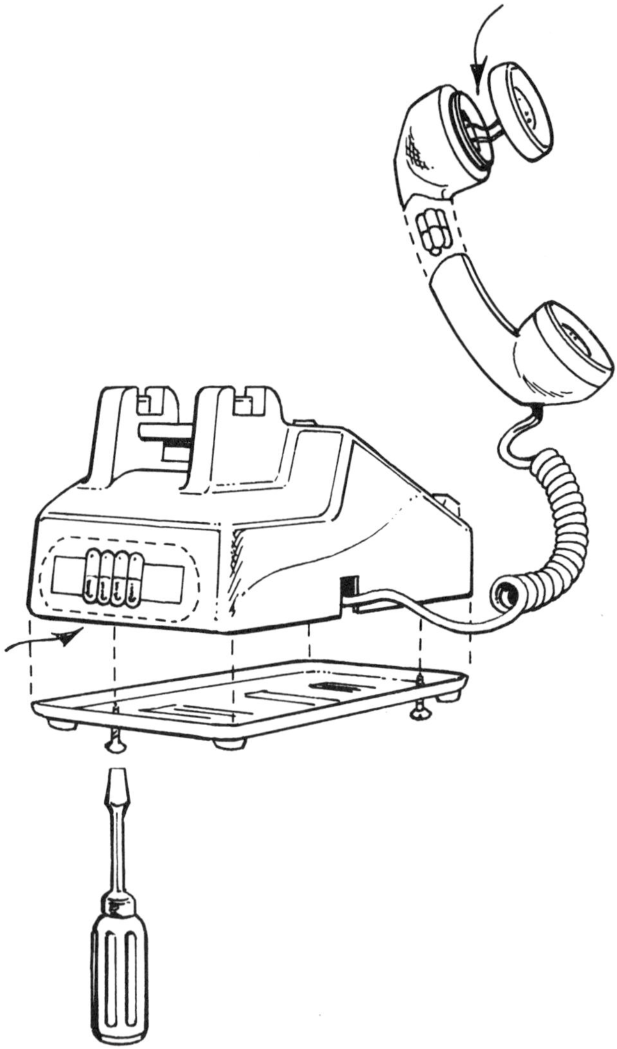

In rain gutters and drain spouts
Inside abandoned plumbing
In attic insulation
Inside or under furnace
In hollowed-out tree
Within fuel of oil heaters
Under lip ring of plastic trash cans
Under tile steps of backyard
Under fence post tops
Inside rabbit hutch
In pay telephone coin return
In telephone base and handle
Behind wall phones
Under telephone name plate
In clothesline pipe
Refrigerator:
- Inside fruit containers
- In eggs
- Inside mayonnaise
- Under food
- Taped under door
- Inside motor compartment
- LSD on food items

Inside garbage disposal unit
Behind electric baseboard heaters
Inside string mop
Under ironing board cover
On bottom of dog food bag
Bottom half of double boiler

BEHIND WALL AND CEILING LIGHT FIXTURES

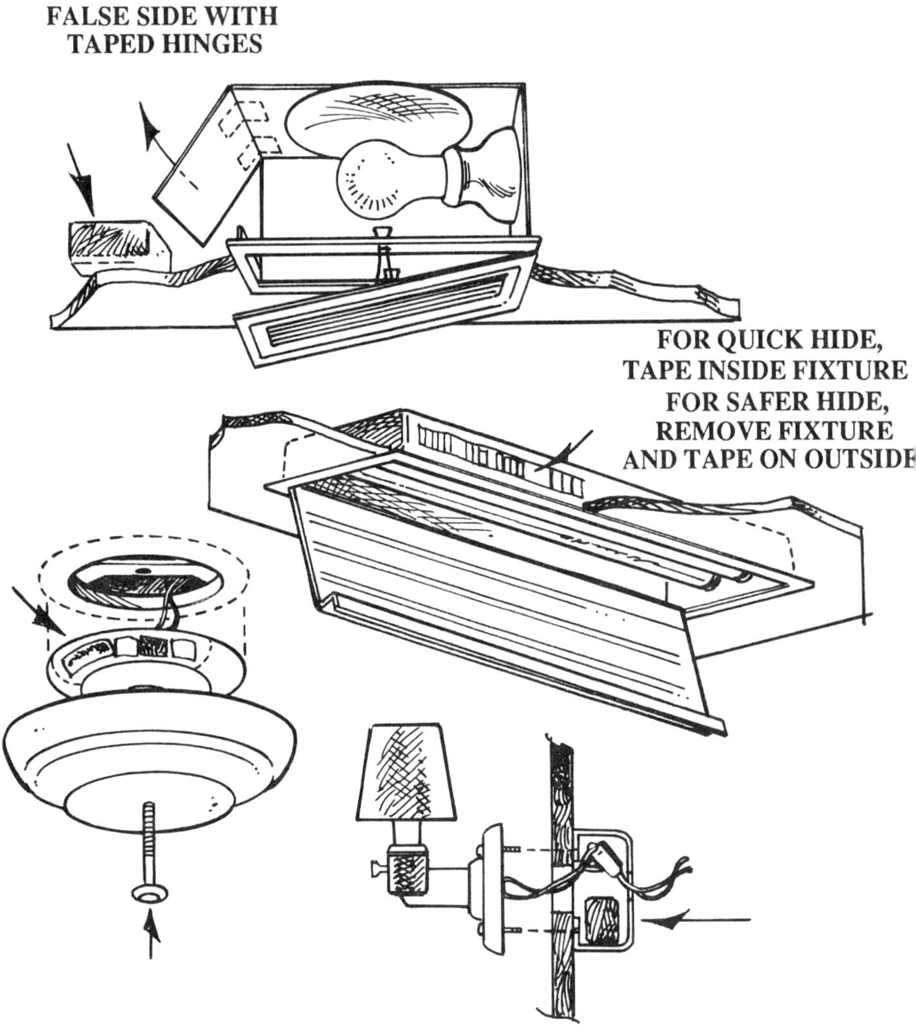

In ironing board legs
Under toaster tray
Inside plastic rolling pin
Inside knife handles
In clock
In hot-air ducts
In stove pipes
In garbage bags
In bromo seltzer, cough syrup, prescription drug bottles
In baked bread, cookies, brownies, and candy bars
Built inside room dividers
Behind kick plates of sink cabinets
In stove insulation, exhausts, and drip pans
Within tea bags
Above acoustic tile ceilings
Inside tinfoil tube
Inside paper towel tube
In salt and pepper shakers
In waxed-paper dispensers
In spice jars
In all kitchen canisters and containers
In hollowed fruits and vegetables
In or on chandelier
Within agitator of clothes washer
On, behind, or above Venetian blinds
In fluorescent light tubes
Behind wall and ceiling light fixtures
Inside light housing
Behind light switches

INSIDE TOILET BOWL FLOAT

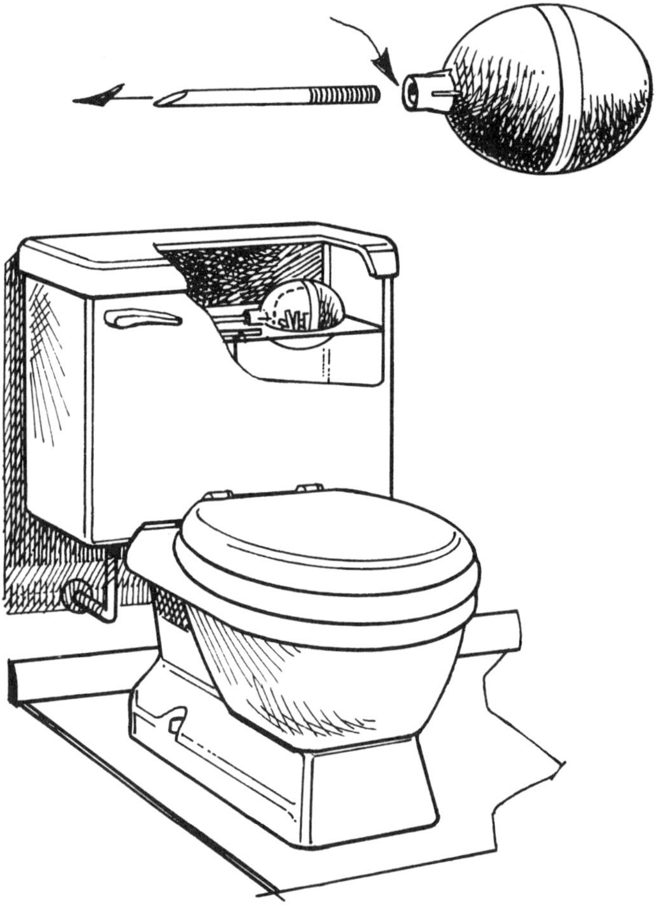

Behind light switches
Inside or behind electric sockets
In removable air-conditioning registers
In range hood and filter
Inside deep well fryers
Behind baseboards
Inside flashlights
Inside douche bags
Within sanitary napkins and in box
In razor blade dispenser
In hollowed-out flashlight batteries
Inside talcum powder, cold cream, and Vaseline containers
In electric toothbrush holder
In toothpaste tubes
In clothes hamper
Hung behind curtains
Inside false ceilings and chimneys
In or behind sink traps
In bases of lamps
Under washbowl, sink, or tub
At bottom of pet litter box
Inside hollow curtain rods, shower curtain rods, and within closet rods
Under false bottom on radiator covers
Inside toilet tanks
Inside toilet bowl float
Taped to top of toilet bowl
Within false aerosol cans

WITHIN HOLLOW SOAP BARS

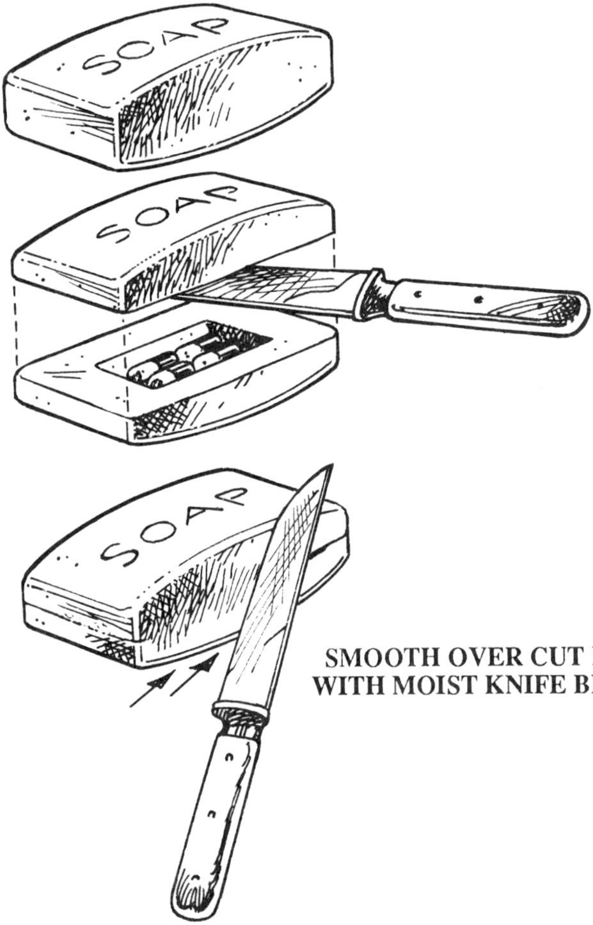

SMOOTH OVER CUT LINE
WITH MOIST KNIFE BLADE

In Bandaids and Bandaid boxes
Inside stick deodorant containers
Within hollow soap bars
Under panel or parquet floors
Inside toilet paper roll
In clothes-pin bag
Inside hollow handle of toilet bowl brush
In after shave, cologne, or cosmetic bottles
Behind and inside medicine cabinets
Inside shaving brush handles
In hair dryer
In shower nozzle head
In razor blade disposal box
In or behind legs of old-style bath tub
Closet clothing:
- In waistbands
- In pens
- In sleeves
- In hatbands
- In shoes
- In gloves

Behind picture frames, posters, and mirrors
In mattresses and box spring frames
Inside pillows
Under carpets
In seams of field cots and hollow cap of cot legs
Inside hassocks
Inside and under wigs
Behind walls

BIBLE (HOLLOW COVER) AND OTHER BOOKS (HOLLOW PAGES)

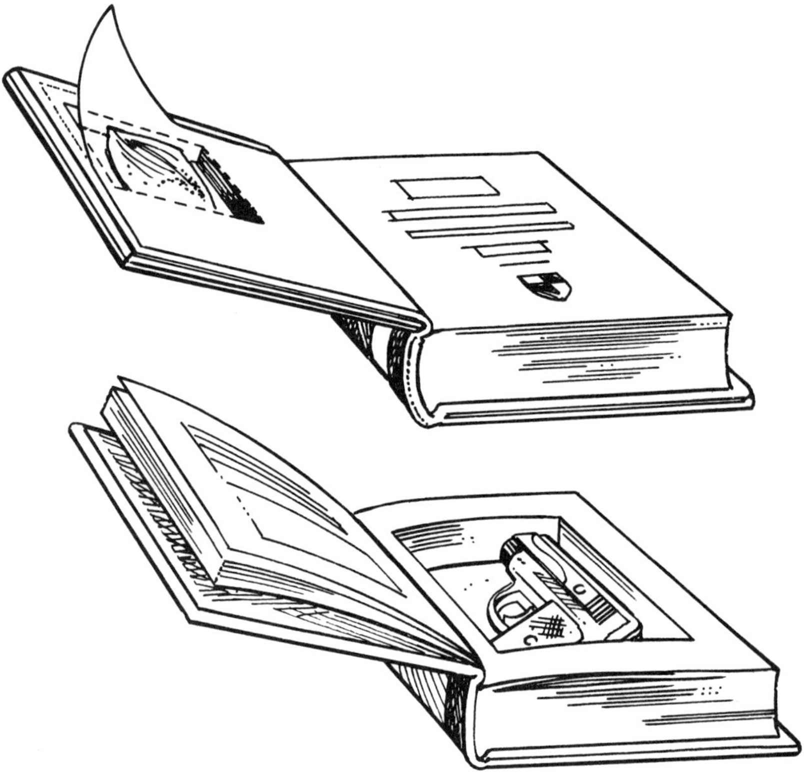

In hollow bedposts
In furniture upholstery
In golf bags
In toys, stuffed animals, and games
Inside child's bank
Taped in dresser and behind drawers
Inside concealed magnet boxes
Inside zippered cushions
Inside pipe rack stand
In false-bottomed baby carriage and cribs
In footlockers
In hem of drapes and curtains
In hidden drawers in tables
Inside letters
In dolls
In art kits
Holy Bible (hollow cover) and other books (hollow pages)
Inside jewelry boxes
Mixed with tobacco
Taped to hat or shoe boxes
LSD on or in blotter
Inside tube and barrel of air rifle
In bird cage
In typewriters and typewriter covers
Inside hollow chess players and boards
Inside hollow canes and umbrellas
In fireplace ash clean-out bin
In drops on graph paper

INSIDE STAIRWAY POSTS

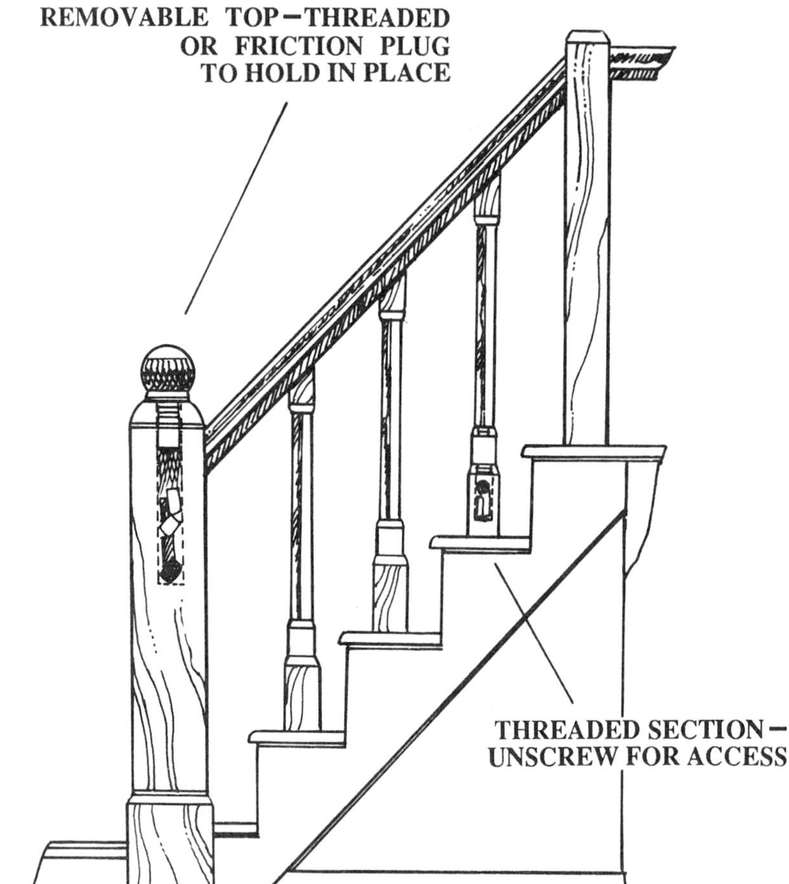

Inside base of rabbit antenna
Inside TV set
Inside TV antenna
Inside altered picture tube or other components
Within hollowed-out pad of paper
In surf boards, skis and other sports equipment
Inside Christmas tree decorations
Inside handle of vacuum cleaners
Inside and behind vacuum cleaner bag
In tool box
In shoe polish container and equipment
In 35 mm film cans
Inside cameras
In record albums
In fish tanks
Inside patch trap of antique rifle
Inside rifle cartridges and shotgun shells
Behind rifle butt plates
Inside carpenter's toolbox
Inside candlestick holders
Inside ceramic and clay figurines
Inside rolled-up newspaper
Inside trophies
In floor drains
In test tubes
Inside crucifix
Inside sealed and opened cigarette packages
Inside stairway posts
Inside transistor radio

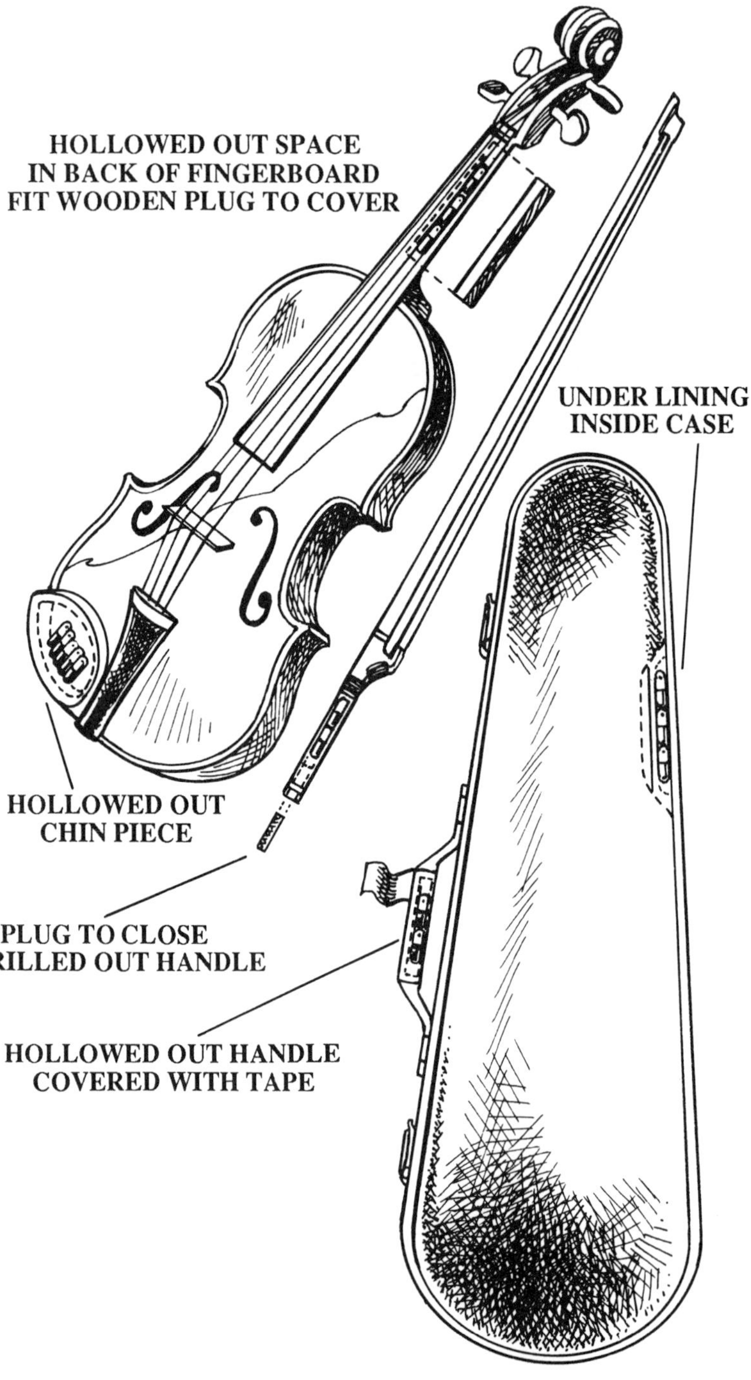
HOLLOWED OUT SPACE
IN BACK OF FINGERBOARD
FIT WOODEN PLUG TO COVER
UNDER LINING
INSIDE CASE
HOLLOWED OUT
CHIN PIECE
PLUG TO CLOSE
DRILLED OUT HANDLE
HOLLOWED OUT HANDLE
COVERED WITH TAPE

Inside speakers
Inside other stereo components
In musical instruments and cases

CONCEALMENT IN AN AUTOMOBILE:

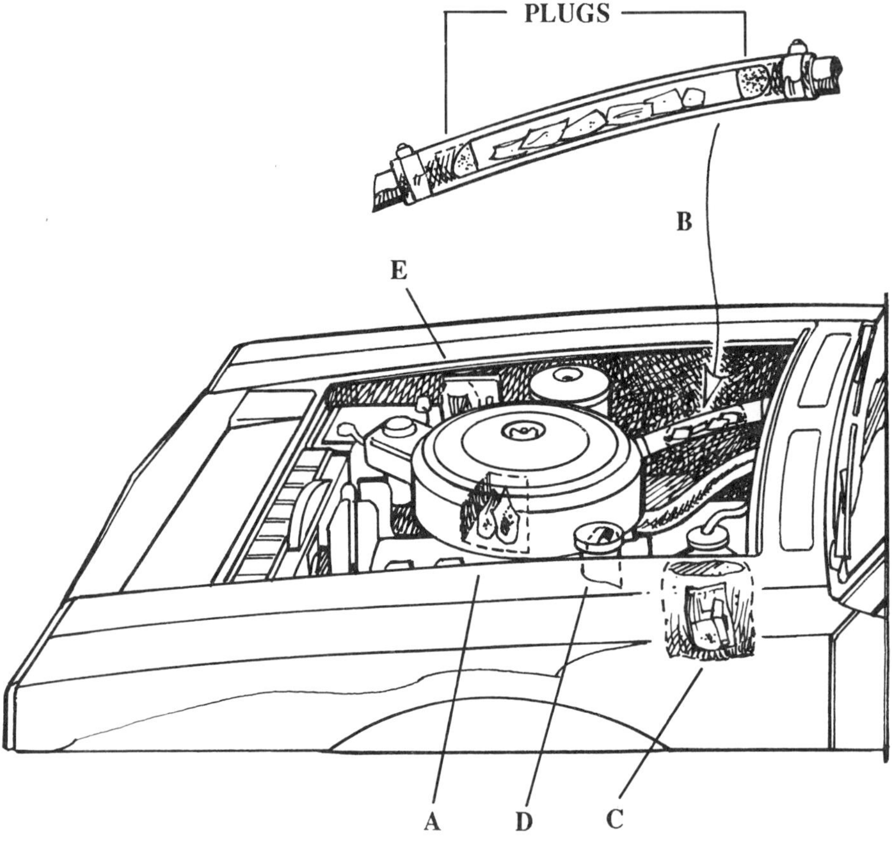

A. IN AIR FILTER

B. IN FALSE HEATER HOSE

C. IN WINDSHIELD WASHER BAG

D. INSIDE OIL CAP

E. IN HOLLOW VOLTAGE REGULATOR

CONCEALMENT IN AN AUTOMOBILE

Inside horn
In air filter
In false heater hose
In heater
In false battery
In oil filter
In windshield washer bag
In carburetor
Inside oil cap
In false dual muffler
In hollow voltage regulator
On top of gas tank (suspended or concealed in compartment)
In 35 mm film cans
Under rocker panels
Tied to axle
Underside of fender
In tail pipe
In insulation under hood

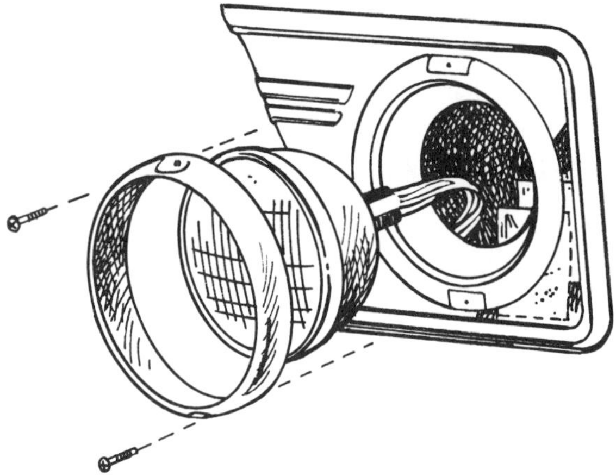

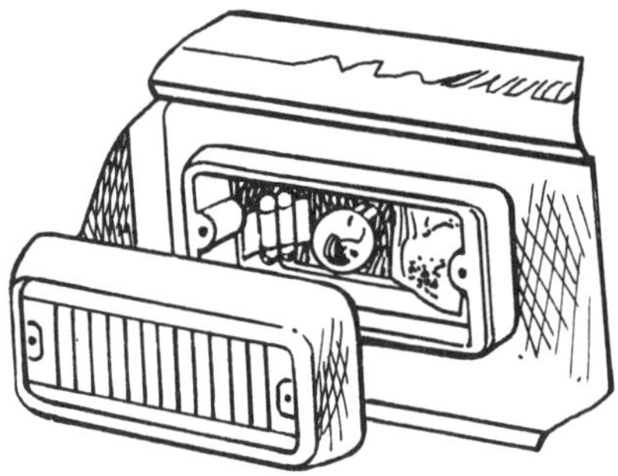

Under chrome
Behind Volkswagen battery box
Inside trunk lids
Inside tubing on roof racks
Inside tubing on surfboard or ski rack
Under tire air valve caps
Taped behind bumper
In antenna base
Taped to rolled-down window
Behind license plates
Attached to frame of car
Behind headlights and taillights
Within hub caps
In picnic jug in trunk
In double roof of surplus police cars
Within spare tire and tire well
In convertible top
In trunk
In fuse box
Under false bottom of trunk beds
In cigarette lighter
Under floorboards
Under front seat
Under back seat
Within vents (air and heater)
In glove compartment -- top of compartment or trap
Within door
Behind radio speaker grill
In shift knob

BEHIND INSTRUMENT PANEL AND
ORNAMENTAL OBJECTS ON DASHBOARD

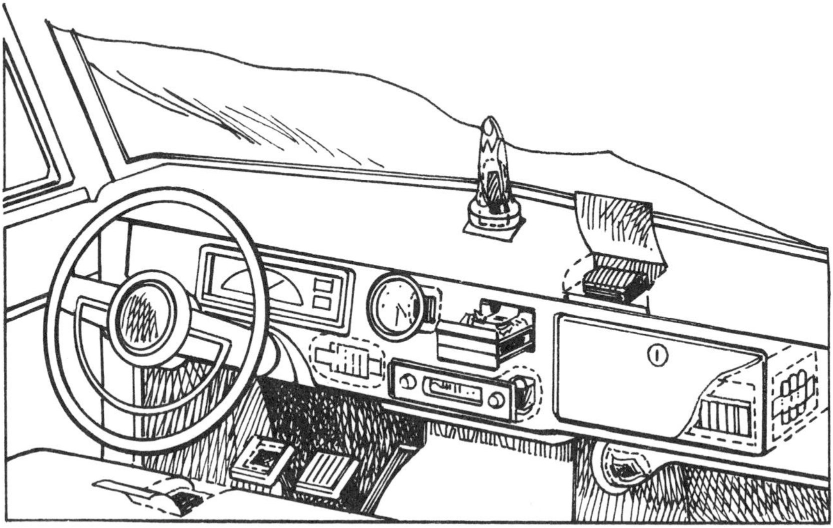

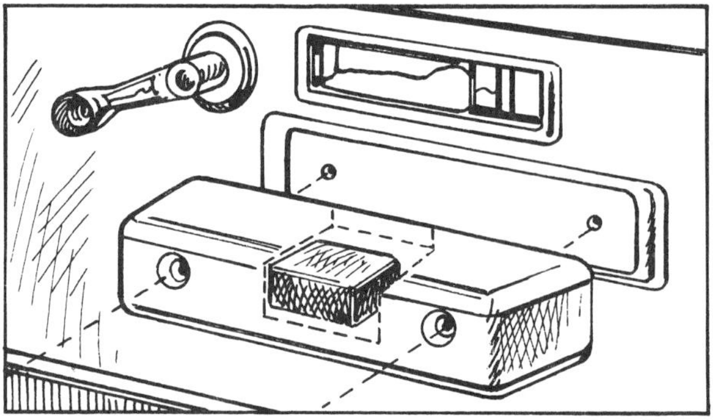

WITHIN ARM RESTS

In steering column
In dome light
In and under ashtrays
Inside key case
In service station travel kits
Under brake and gas pedals
In or behind sun visors
Under carpet
Behind or within false radio
Inside a hide-a-key container
Pill vials
Under floor mats
Within upholstery
Behind instrumental panel
Under ornamental objects on dashboard
Within compartments under floor of older VWs and Jeeps
Inside floor consoles
Inside dash knobs
Within arm rests
Inside flashlight
Inside toolbox
Inside light sockets

MOTORCYCLES:

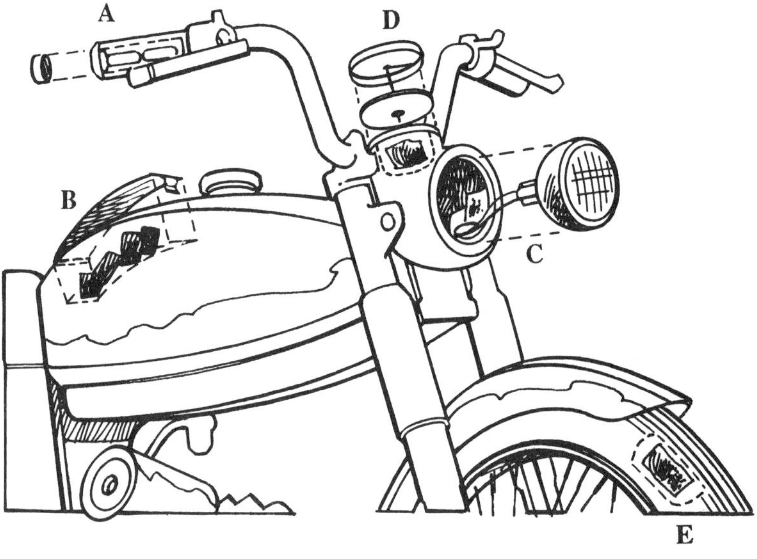

A. INSIDE HANDLEBAR TUBING

B. COMPARTMENT IN CUSTOM GAS TANK

C. BEHIND HEADLIGHT

D. BEHIND INSTRUMENT GAUGES

E. INSIDE TIRES

CONCEALMENT ON A MOTORCYCLE

Behind taillights
Under seats
Inside handlebar tubing
Inside battery box
In toolbox
Rolled up inside sleeping bag or other carried items
Concealed compartment in custom gas tank
Inside lining of motorcycle helmet
In concealed pockets in padded clothing
Behind headlight
Behind instrument gauges
Inside tires

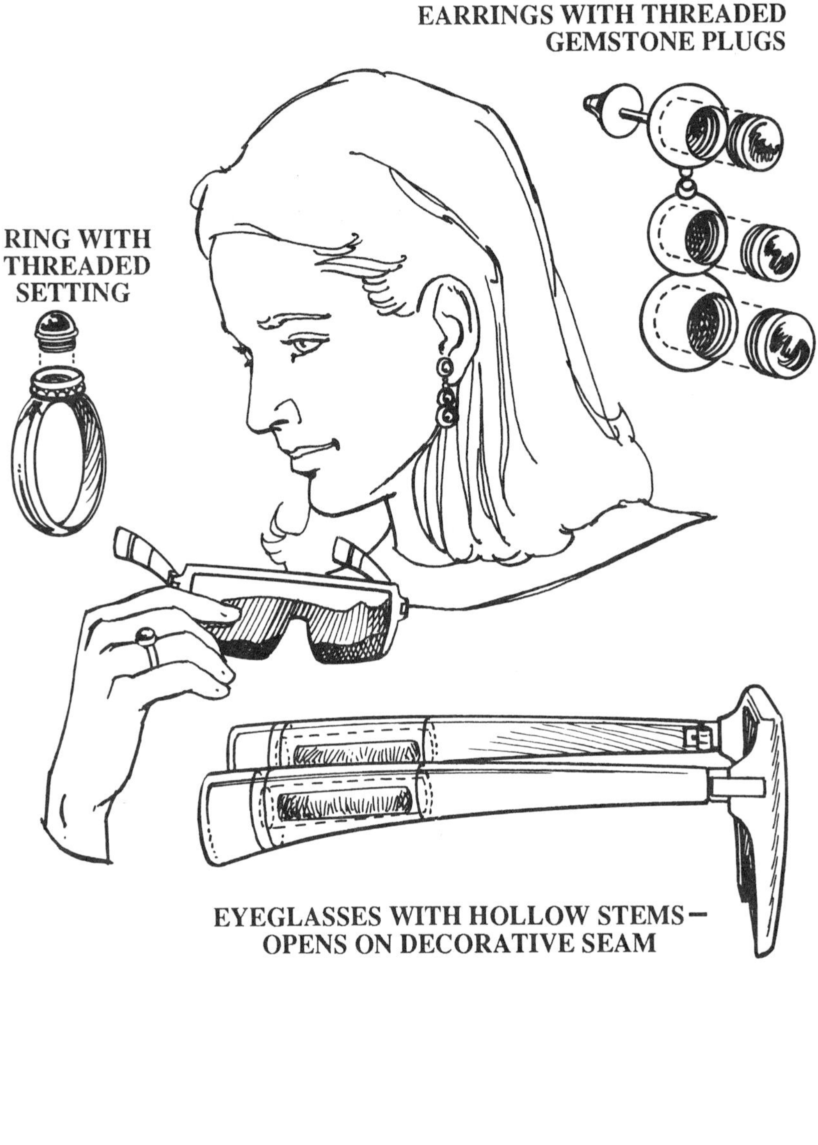
EARRINGS WITH THREADED
GEMSTONE PLUGS
RING WITH
THREADED
SETTING
EYEGLASSES WITH HOLLOW STEMS –
OPENS ON DECORATIVE SEAM

CONCEALMENT ON THE PERSON

Inside false caps on teeth
Swallowed with string tied to teeth
Under false teeth
Loose in mouth
Behind or in ears
In glass eyes
In nose
Taped under breasts
In brassiere
Under Bandaids and bandages
Within rectum
Within vagina
Between cheeks of buttocks
Under foreskin of penis
Inside feces bag
In false leg, arm, foot, etc.
In or behind womens' hair barrettes
Under processed hair, hair buns, or wigs
In hearing aids mounted on eyeglasses or within ears
In earrings

IN HOLLOW END OF CANE OR UMBRELLA

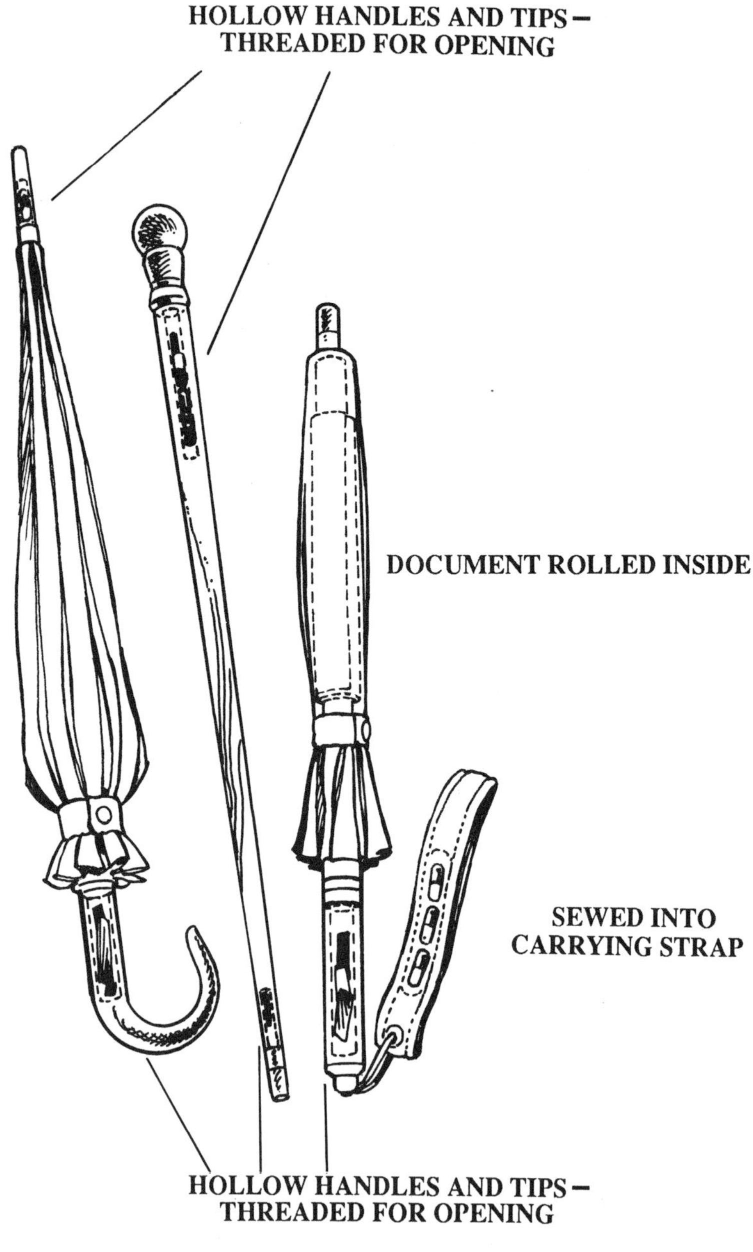

In rings
Inside neck and wrist lockets, bracelets, and charms
Inside ID bracelets
In plaster or plastic casts

Under hatbands
In hats
Under military cap insignia
Under lapel and shoulder patches
Behind campaign ribbons and uniform brass
Hashish in love beads
In fountain pens
In money belts, slit or zippered
In tie pins, clasps, and cuff links
In lining of clothing
Within false buttons
Under lapels of jacket and coats
Inside back of watch
In pockets
In eyeglass case
In corsets
In tie knot of tie and handkerchiefs
Jockstraps
Wallet
In hollow belt buckles
Inside fly flap of trousers
Pinned to shorts
In swimming trunks
In male or female girdle

CONCEALMENT ON THE PERSON:

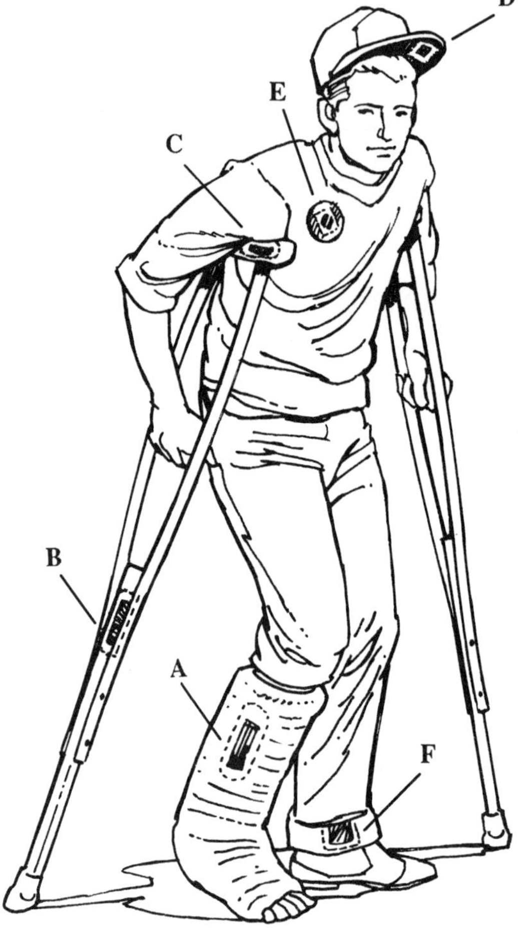

A. IN PLASTER CAST

B. IN NON-SUPPORTING SECTION OF CRUTCH

C. IN ARM PAD OF CRUTCH (TAPED OVER)

D. IN HAT

E. IN BUTTON

F. IN CUFF

Inside cuffs and waistbands
In socks and shoes
In baby's diapers
In lipstick tube
In tobacco tins and pouches
In cigarette package
In cigarette lighters
Inside hollowed-out crutches
In hollow end of cane or umbrella
Inside feces bag
In Thermos jug cavity or lining
In canteens
In addressed envelopes
Within liners of luggage